CALORIC DEFICIT
WEIGHT LOSS
Diet

Rapid Weight Loss
for Seniors

FRANK A. KELEMEN

CALORIC DEFICIT Diet
for Seniors

Contents

CALORIC DEFICIT Diet

Weight Loss Recipes for Seniors

Benefits

1. Gradual Weight Loss:

   - The moderate calorie deficit promotes steady, sustainable weight loss without drastic measures.

   - This approach is gentler on the body, which is particularly important for seniors.

2. Muscle Preservation:

   - The high-protein content helps maintain muscle mass during weight loss.

   - This is crucial for seniors to maintain strength, balance, and overall functionality.

3. Improved Metabolic Health:

   - Weight loss can lead to better insulin sensitivity and improved blood sugar control.

   - May help in managing or preventing type 2 diabetes, a common concern in older adults.

4. Reduced Inflammation:

   - The diet's focus on whole, nutrient-dense foods can help reduce systemic inflammation.

   - This may alleviate symptoms of inflammatory conditions common in seniors, such as arthritis.

5. Better Cardiovascular Health:

   - Weight loss and the heart-healthy food choices can improve blood pressure and cholesterol levels.

- This reduces the risk of heart disease and stroke.

6. Increased Mobility:

   - Losing excess weight reduces stress on joints, potentially improving mobility and reducing pain.

   - This can lead to increased physical activity and better overall quality of life.

7. Enhanced Digestive Health:

   - The high-fiber content promotes regular bowel movements and a healthy gut microbiome.

   - This can alleviate common digestive issues in seniors like constipation.

8. Improved Nutrient Absorption:

   - The nutrient-dense nature of the diet ensures seniors get essential vitamins and minerals.

   - This is particularly important as nutrient absorption often decreases with age.

9. Better Sleep Quality:

   - Weight loss and improved diet quality are associated with better sleep patterns.

   - Good sleep is crucial for cognitive function and overall health in seniors.

10. Mood Enhancement:

   - Balanced nutrition and weight loss can positively impact mood and reduce the risk of depression.

   - The social aspect of preparing meals can also combat feelings of isolation.

11. Cognitive Benefits:

   - The diet's emphasis on foods rich in omega-3 fatty acids and antioxidants may support brain health.

   - This could potentially slow cognitive decline associated with aging.

12. Increased Energy Levels:

   - Balanced meals provide steady energy throughout the day.

   - Weight loss itself often leads to increased energy and vitality.

13. Improved Immune Function:

   - A nutrient-rich diet supports the immune system, which is particularly important for seniors.

14. Better Management of Chronic Conditions:

   - Weight loss and improved nutrition can help manage conditions like osteoarthritis, hypertension, and sleep apnea.

15. Reduced Medication Dependence:

   - As health improves, there may be a reduced need for certain medications, always under doctor's supervision.

Remember, while these benefits are significant, it's crucial for seniors to consult with their healthcare provider before starting any new diet plan, especially if they have existing health conditions or are on medications.

Rate of Weigh Loss

When discussing the rate of weight loss for this caloric deficit meal plan, it's important to note that individual results can vary based on factors such as starting weight, body composition, activity level, and metabolic rate. However, I can provide an estimate based on the caloric deficit created by this meal plan.

Rate of Weight Loss for this Caloric Deficit Meal Plan

General Expectation:

This meal plan is designed to create a moderate caloric deficit, aiming for a safe and sustainable weight loss rate of about 0.5 to 1 pound (0.23 to 0.45 kg) per week for most seniors. This rate is considered healthy and manageable, especially for older adults.

Breakdown by Week:

Week 1

- Expected weight loss: 0.5 to 1 pound (0.23 to 0.45 kg)

- Note: Initial weight loss might be higher due to water weight loss

Week 2

- Expected weight loss: 0.5 to 1 pound (0.23 to 0.45 kg)

- Cumulative loss: 1 to 2 pounds (0.45 to 0.9 kg)

Week 3

- Expected weight loss: 0.5 to 1 pound (0.23 to 0.45 kg)

- Cumulative loss: 1.5 to 3 pounds (0.68 to 1.36 kg)

Week 4

- Expected weight loss: 0.5 to 1 pound (0.23 to 0.45 kg)

- Cumulative loss: 2 to 4 pounds (0.9 to 1.8 kg)

Total Expected Weight Loss After 30 Days:

2 to 4 pounds (0.9 to 1.8 kg)

Important Considerations:

1. Individual Variation: Some seniors may lose weight more slowly or quickly depending on their unique circumstances.

2. Non-Linear Progress: Weight loss is often not linear. Some weeks may show more loss than others.

3. Body Composition Changes: The scale might not reflect all progress as muscle preservation can offset fat loss.

4. Water Weight Fluctuations: Daily weight can fluctuate due to hydration levels, sodium intake, and other factors.

5. Beyond the Scale: Improvements in energy levels, mobility, and overall health may be noticeable even if weight loss is modest.

6. Plateaus: It's normal for weight loss to slow or stall temporarily. Consistency is key.

7. Adjustment Period: The body may take some time to adjust to the new eating pattern, which can affect initial weight loss rates.

8. Safety First: This moderate rate of weight loss is designed to be safe and sustainable for seniors, prioritizing overall health over rapid weight loss.

Remember, the goal of this meal plan is not just weight loss, but overall health improvement. Seniors should focus on how they feel, their energy levels, and other health markers in addition to the number on the scale. Always consult with a healthcare provider to ensure the diet and weight loss rate are appropriate for individual health conditions and needs.

30 Day CALORIC DEFICIT Diet - Recipes and Meal Plan

Each day provides a balance of protein, complex carbohydrates, and healthy fats, while maintaining a calorie deficit for weight loss.

The meals are designed to be easy to prepare and nutrient-dense, which is especially important for seniors.

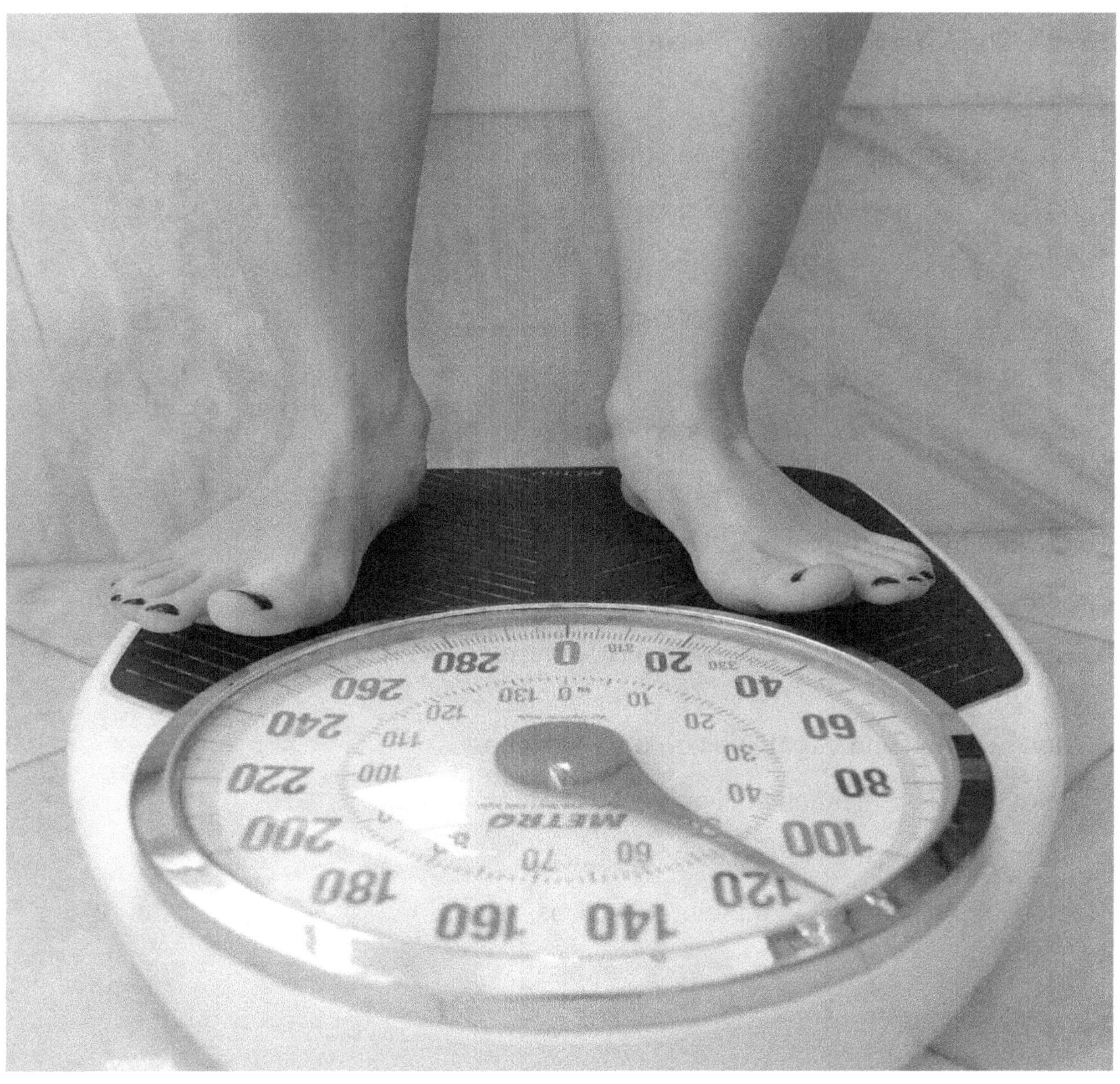

Day 1

Breakfast: Oatmeal with Berries

Recipe:

1. Combine 1/2 cup rolled oats with 1 cup unsweetened almond milk in a microwave-safe bowl.

2. Microwave for 2 minutes, stirring halfway through.

3. Top with 1/2 cup mixed berries and 1 tbsp chopped walnuts.

Macros: 290 calories, 11g protein, 42g carbs, 10g fat

Lunch: Greek Yogurt Chicken Salad

Recipe:

1. Mix 3 oz cooked, diced chicken breast with 1/4 cup Greek yogurt.

2. Add 1/4 cup diced celery, 1/4 cup diced apple, and 1 tbsp chopped pecans.

3. Serve on a bed of mixed greens.

Macros: 280 calories, 32g protein, 14g carbs, 12g fat

Dinner: Baked Salmon with Roasted Vegetables

Recipe:

1. Preheat oven to 400°F (200°C).

2. Season 4 oz salmon fillet with herbs and lemon juice.

3. Toss 1 cup mixed vegetables (broccoli, carrots, zucchini) with olive oil and seasonings.

4. Place salmon and vegetables on a baking sheet.

5. Bake for 12-15 minutes until salmon is cooked through.

6. Serve with 1/2 small baked sweet potato.

Macros: 350 calories, 28g protein, 25g carbs, 18g fat

Day 2

Breakfast: Veggie Egg Scramble

Recipe:

1. Whisk 2 eggs in a bowl.

2. Sauté 1/4 cup diced bell peppers and 1/4 cup diced onions in a non-stick pan.

3. Add 1/2 cup spinach and cook until wilted.

4. Pour in whisked eggs and scramble until cooked.

5. Serve with 1 slice whole grain toast.

Macros: 270 calories, 18g protein, 22g carbs, 14g fat

Lunch: Lentil Soup

Recipe:

1. In a pot, sauté 1/4 cup each of diced onions, carrots, and celery.

2. Add 1/4 cup dry lentils, 1 cup water, and seasonings.

3. Simmer for 20-25 minutes until lentils are tender.

4. Serve with 1 small whole grain roll.

Macros: 300 calories, 16g protein, 48g carbs, 6g fat

Dinner: Turkey Meatballs with Zucchini Noodles

Recipe:

1. Mix 3 oz lean ground turkey with breadcrumbs, egg, and seasonings.

2. Form into meatballs and bake at 375°F (190°C) for 15-20 minutes.

3. Spiralize 1 medium zucchini to make noodles.

4. Sauté zucchini noodles lightly.

5. Serve meatballs over zucchini noodles with 1/4 cup marinara sauce and 1 tbsp grated Parmesan.

Macros: 320 calories, 32g protein, 18g carbs, 15g fat

Day 3

Breakfast: Cottage Cheese with Fruit

Recipe:

1. In a bowl, combine 1/2 cup low-fat cottage cheese with 1/2 cup mixed berries.

2. Sprinkle 1 tbsp chia seeds and 1/4 cup granola on top.

Macros: 280 calories, 19g protein, 35g carbs, 9g fat

Lunch: Tuna Avocado Wrap

Recipe:

1. Mash 1/4 avocado in a bowl.

2. Mix in 3 oz canned tuna (drained) and 1/4 cup diced cucumber.

3. Spread the mixture on a whole wheat tortilla and roll up.

Macros: 310 calories, 28g protein, 25g carbs, 13g fat

Dinner: Slow Cooker Chicken and Vegetable Stew

Recipe:

1. In a slow cooker, combine 4 oz diced chicken breast, 1 cup mixed vegetables (carrots, celery, onions, peas), and 1/2 cup low-sodium chicken broth.

2. Add herbs and spices to taste.

3. Cook on low for 6-8 hours or on high for 3-4 hours.

Macros: 280 calories, 35g protein, 20g carbs, 6g fat

Certainly. Let's continue with the next three days of the meal plan:

Day 4

Breakfast: Whole Grain Toast with Avocado and Egg

Recipe:

1. Toast 1 slice of whole grain bread.

2. Mash 1/4 avocado and spread on toast.

3. Top with 1 poached egg and a sprinkle of salt and pepper.

Macros: 260 calories, 13g protein, 20g carbs, 16g fat

Lunch: Quinoa and Black Bean Bowl

Recipe:

1. Cook 1/4 cup quinoa according to package instructions.

2. Mix with 1/4 cup canned black beans (drained and rinsed).

3. Add 1/4 cup diced tomatoes, 1/4 cup diced bell peppers, and 1 tbsp chopped cilantro.

4. Dress with 1 tsp olive oil and lime juice.

Macros: 300 calories, 12g protein, 50g carbs, 8g fat

Dinner: Grilled Chicken with Roasted Sweet Potato and Broccoli

Recipe:

1. Season 4 oz chicken breast and grill until cooked through.

2. Cut 1 small sweet potato into cubes, toss with 1 tsp olive oil and roast at 400°F for 20-25 minutes.

3. Steam 1 cup broccoli florets.

Macros: 340 calories, 35g protein, 30g carbs, 9g fat

Day 5

Breakfast: Greek Yogurt Parfait

Recipe:

1. Layer 1/2 cup Greek yogurt with 1/4 cup mixed berries and 2 tbsp low-fat granola.

2. Drizzle with 1 tsp honey.

Macros: 240 calories, 20g protein, 30g carbs, 5g fat

Lunch: Spinach and Chickpea Salad

Recipe:

1. Mix 2 cups spinach with 1/4 cup canned chickpeas (drained and rinsed).

2. Add 1/4 cup diced cucumber, 2 tbsp feta cheese, and 5 halved cherry tomatoes.

3. Dress with 1 tsp olive oil and balsamic vinegar.

Macros: 250 calories, 12g protein, 25g carbs, 13g fat

Dinner: Baked Cod with Quinoa and Roasted Vegetables

Recipe:

1. Season 4 oz cod fillet and bake at 375°F for 15-20 minutes.

2. Cook 1/4 cup quinoa according to package instructions.

3. Roast 1 cup mixed vegetables (zucchini, bell peppers, onions) at 400°F for 20 minutes.

Macros: 320 calories, 30g protein, 35g carbs, 7g fat

Day 6

Breakfast: Banana Peanut Butter Smoothie

Recipe:

1. Blend 1 small banana, 1 cup unsweetened almond milk, 1 tbsp peanut butter, and 1/2 scoop vanilla protein powder.

2. Add ice cubes if desired.

Macros: 280 calories, 18g protein, 35g carbs, 11g fat

Lunch: Turkey and Avocado Lettuce Wraps

Recipe:

1. Layer 3 oz sliced turkey breast, 1/4 sliced avocado, 2 slices tomato, and 1 leaf lettuce on each of 2 large lettuce leaves.

2. Roll up and secure with toothpicks if needed.

Macros: 260 calories, 25g protein, 10g carbs, 15g fat

Dinner: Lentil and Vegetable Curry

Recipe:

1. Sauté 1/4 cup each of diced onions, carrots, and bell peppers.

2. Add 1/4 cup cooked lentils, 1/4 cup coconut milk, and 1 tbsp curry powder.

3. Simmer for 10 minutes.

4. Serve over 1/4 cup cooked brown rice.

Macros: 340 calories, 14g protein, 50g carbs, 12g fat

Day 7

Breakfast: Whole Grain Waffle with Almond Butter and Banana

Recipe:

1. Toast 1 whole grain waffle.

2. Spread 1 tbsp almond butter on the waffle.

3. Top with 1/2 sliced banana.

Macros: 280 calories, 10g protein, 40g carbs, 12g fat

Lunch: Mediterranean Chickpea Salad

Recipe:

1. Mix 1/4 cup canned chickpeas (drained and rinsed) with 1/4 cup diced cucumber, 1/4 cup diced tomatoes, and 2 tbsp diced red onion.

2. Add 1 tbsp crumbled feta cheese and 5 halved kalamata olives.

3. Dress with 1 tsp olive oil and 1 tsp lemon juice.

4. Sprinkle with dried oregano.

Macros: 300 calories, 15g protein, 35g carbs, 14g fat

Dinner: Grilled Tilapia with Quinoa and Asparagus

Recipe:

1. Season 4 oz tilapia fillet with lemon juice, garlic, and herbs.

2. Grill for 3-4 minutes per side until cooked through.

3. Cook 1/4 cup quinoa according to package instructions.

4. Steam 1 cup asparagus spears.

Macros: 330 calories, 35g protein, 30g carbs, 8g fat

Day 8

Breakfast: Spinach and Mushroom Frittata

Recipe:

1. Whisk 2 eggs with 1 tbsp milk.

2. Sauté 1/4 cup sliced mushrooms and 1/2 cup spinach in a small oven-safe pan.

3. Pour egg mixture over vegetables and cook until edges set.

4. Finish under the broiler for 2-3 minutes.

Macros: 250 calories, 20g protein, 15g carbs, 15g fat

Lunch: Whole Grain Pita with Hummus and Vegetables

Recipe:

1. Spread 2 tbsp hummus inside a whole grain pita half.

2. Fill with 1/4 cup sliced cucumber, 1/4 cup sliced bell peppers, and 1/4 cup shredded carrots.

Macros: 280 calories, 12g protein, 40g carbs, 10g fat

Dinner: Slow Cooker Beef and Vegetable Stew

Recipe:

1. In a slow cooker, combine 3 oz lean beef cubes, 1 cup mixed vegetables (carrots, celery, onions, peas), 1/2 cup low-sodium beef broth, and herbs.

2. Cook on low for 6-8 hours or on high for 3-4 hours.

Macros: 350 calories, 30g protein, 25g carbs, 15g fat

Day 9

Breakfast: Overnight Chia Seed Pudding

Recipe:

1. In a jar, mix 2 tbsp chia seeds with 1/2 cup unsweetened almond milk and 1 tsp honey.

2. Refrigerate overnight.

3. In the morning, top with 1/4 cup mixed berries and 1 tbsp sliced almonds.

Macros: 260 calories, 12g protein, 35g carbs, 12g fat

Lunch: Tuna and White Bean Salad

Recipe:

1. Mix 3 oz canned tuna (drained) with 1/4 cup canned white beans (drained and rinsed).

2. Add 1/4 cup diced celery, 1 tbsp diced red onion, and 1 tsp olive oil.

3. Season with lemon juice and herbs.

4. Serve over a bed of mixed greens.

Macros: 290 calories, 30g protein, 20g carbs, 10g fat

Dinner: Baked Chicken Breast with Sweet Potato and Green Beans

Recipe:

1. Season 4 oz chicken breast and bake at 375°F for 20-25 minutes.

2. Bake 1/2 small sweet potato at the same time.

3. Steam 1 cup green beans.

Macros: 340 calories, 35g protein, 30g carbs, 8g fat

Day 10

Breakfast: Greek Yogurt with Honey and Walnuts

Recipe:

1. Mix 3/4 cup Greek yogurt with 1 tsp honey.

2. Top with 1 tbsp chopped walnuts and 1/4 cup sliced strawberries.

Macros: 270 calories, 20g protein, 25g carbs, 14g fat

Lunch: Lentil and Vegetable Soup

Recipe:

1. In a pot, sauté 1/4 cup each of diced onions, carrots, and celery.

2. Add 1/4 cup dry lentils, 1 cup vegetable broth, and seasonings.

3. Simmer for 20-25 minutes until lentils are tender.

Macros: 280 calories, 15g protein, 45g carbs, 5g fat

Dinner: Grilled Salmon with Brown Rice and Broccoli

Recipe:

1. Season 4 oz salmon fillet and grill for 4-5 minutes per side.

2. Cook 1/4 cup brown rice according to package instructions.

3. Steam 1 cup broccoli florets.

Macros: 360 calories, 30g protein, 35g carbs, 12g fat

Day 11

Breakfast: Whole Grain Toast with Avocado and Smoked Salmon

Recipe:

1. Toast 1 slice of whole grain bread.

2. Mash 1/4 avocado and spread on toast.

3. Top with 2 oz smoked salmon and a squeeze of lemon juice.

Macros: 290 calories, 18g protein, 20g carbs, 18g fat

Lunch: Quinoa and Roasted Vegetable Bowl

Recipe:

1. Cook 1/4 cup quinoa according to package instructions.

2. Roast 1 cup mixed vegetables (zucchini, bell peppers, onions) at 400°F for 20 minutes.

3. Combine quinoa and vegetables, dress with 1 tsp olive oil and balsamic vinegar.

Macros: 300 calories, 12g protein, 45g carbs, 10g fat

Dinner: Turkey Meatloaf with Cauliflower Mash

Recipe:

1. Mix 4 oz ground turkey with 1 tbsp breadcrumbs, 1 tbsp beaten egg, and seasonings.

2. Shape into a loaf and bake at 350°F for 25-30 minutes.

3. Steam 1 cup cauliflower florets and mash with 1 tbsp Greek yogurt.

Macros: 330 calories, 35g protein, 20g carbs, 14g fat

Certainly, I'll continue with the next set of days in the same format.

Day 12

Breakfast: Banana Oatmeal Pancakes

Recipe:

1. Blend 1/3 cup rolled oats, 1 small banana, 1 egg, and 1/4 tsp baking powder.

2. Cook in a non-stick pan, making 2-3 small pancakes.

3. Top with 1 tsp maple syrup.

Macros: 280 calories, 12g protein, 45g carbs, 8g fat

Lunch: Grilled Chicken Caesar Salad (with light dressing)

Recipe:

1. Grill 3 oz chicken breast and slice.

2. Toss 2 cups romaine lettuce with 1 tbsp light Caesar dressing.

3. Add grilled chicken and 1 tbsp grated Parmesan cheese.

Macros: 310 calories, 35g protein, 10g carbs, 16g fat

Dinner: Baked Cod with Ratatouille

Recipe:

1. Season 4 oz cod fillet and bake at 375°F for 15-20 minutes.

2. For ratatouille, sauté 1 cup mixed vegetables (eggplant, zucchini, tomatoes, bell peppers) with herbs.

Macros: 320 calories, 30g protein, 25g carbs, 10g fat

Day 13

Breakfast: Cottage Cheese with Peaches and Almonds

Recipe:

1. Combine 1/2 cup low-fat cottage cheese with 1/2 cup sliced peaches.

2. Top with 1 tbsp sliced almonds.

Macros: 260 calories, 20g protein, 25g carbs, 10g fat

Lunch: Turkey and Avocado Sandwich on Whole Grain Bread

Recipe:

1. Spread 1/4 mashed avocado on 1 slice whole grain bread.

2. Add 3 oz sliced turkey breast, 1 slice tomato, and lettuce.

3. Top with another slice of bread.

Macros: 320 calories, 25g protein, 30g carbs, 14g fat

Dinner: Vegetarian Chili with Mixed Beans

Recipe:

1. Sauté 1/4 cup each of diced onions, bell peppers, and carrots.

2. Add 1/2 cup mixed beans, 1/4 cup crushed tomatoes, and chili seasonings.

3. Simmer for 15-20 minutes.

Macros: 300 calories, 18g protein, 45g carbs, 6g fat

Day 14

Breakfast: Scrambled Eggs with Spinach and Feta

Recipe:

1. Whisk 2 eggs and cook in a non-stick pan.

2. Add 1/2 cup spinach and 1 tbsp crumbled feta cheese.

3. Serve with 1 slice whole grain toast.

Macros: 270 calories, 20g protein, 10g carbs, 18g fat

Lunch: Greek Salad with Grilled Chicken

Recipe:

1. Grill 3 oz chicken breast and slice.

2. Toss 2 cups mixed greens with 1/4 cup diced cucumber, 1/4 cup diced tomatoes, 5 kalamata olives, and 1 tbsp crumbled feta.

3. Add grilled chicken and dress with 1 tsp olive oil and lemon juice.

Macros: 310 calories, 30g protein, 15g carbs, 16g fat

Dinner: Baked Trout with Roasted Brussels Sprouts and Quinoa

Recipe:

1. Season 4 oz trout fillet and bake at 375°F for 12-15 minutes.

2. Roast 1 cup halved Brussels sprouts at 400°F for 20 minutes.

3. Cook 1/4 cup quinoa according to package instructions.

Macros: 350 calories, 35g protein, 30g carbs, 12g fat

Day 15

Breakfast: Whole Grain English Muffin with Peanut Butter and Banana

Recipe:

1. Toast 1 whole grain English muffin.

2. Spread 1 tbsp peanut butter on each half.

3. Top with 1/2 sliced banana.

Macros: 290 calories, 12g protein, 40g carbs, 12g fat

Lunch: Lentil and Vegetable Curry over Brown Rice

Recipe:

1. Sauté 1/4 cup each of diced onions, carrots, and bell peppers.

2. Add 1/4 cup cooked lentils, 1/4 cup light coconut milk, and 1 tsp curry powder.

3. Simmer for 10 minutes and serve over 1/4 cup cooked brown rice.

Macros: 320 calories, 15g protein, 50g carbs, 8g fat

Dinner: Grilled Pork Tenderloin with Roasted Sweet Potato and Asparagus

Recipe:

1. Grill 3 oz seasoned pork tenderloin.

2. Roast 1/2 small sweet potato, cubed, at 400°F for 20 minutes.

3. Grill or roast 1 cup asparagus spears.

Macros: 340 calories, 35g protein, 30g carbs, 10g fat

Certainly, I'll continue with the next set of days in the same detailed format.

Day 16

Breakfast: Yogurt and Berry Smoothie Bowl

Recipe:

1. Blend 1/2 cup Greek yogurt, 1/2 cup mixed berries, and 1/4 cup unsweetened almond milk.

2. Pour into a bowl and top with 1 tbsp chia seeds and 1 tbsp sliced almonds.

Macros: 270 calories, 20g protein, 30g carbs, 12g fat

Lunch: Tuna Niçoise Salad

Recipe:

1. Mix 3 oz canned tuna with 1 cup mixed greens, 1/4 cup steamed green beans, 5 halved cherry tomatoes, 5 sliced olives, and 1 small boiled potato (cubed).

2. Dress with 1 tsp olive oil and 1 tsp lemon juice.

Macros: 300 calories, 28g protein, 25g carbs, 13g fat

Dinner: Veggie and Tofu Stir-Fry with Brown Rice

Recipe:

1. Stir-fry 3 oz cubed firm tofu with 1 cup mixed vegetables (broccoli, carrots, snap peas) in 1 tsp oil.

2. Season with low-sodium soy sauce and ginger.

3. Serve over 1/4 cup cooked brown rice.

Macros: 320 calories, 20g protein, 40g carbs, 12g fat

Day 17

Breakfast: Whole Grain Toast with Ricotta and Figs

Recipe:

1. Toast 1 slice whole grain bread.

2. Spread with 2 tbsp low-fat ricotta cheese.

3. Top with 2 sliced fresh figs and a drizzle of honey.

Macros: 250 calories, 12g protein, 40g carbs, 6g fat

Lunch: Chicken and Quinoa Stuffed Bell Peppers

Recipe:

1. Mix 2 oz cooked, diced chicken with 1/4 cup cooked quinoa and 2 tbsp diced tomatoes.

2. Stuff mixture into 1 halved bell pepper.

3. Bake at 375°F for 20 minutes.

Macros: 280 calories, 25g protein, 30g carbs, 8g fat

Dinner: Baked Salmon with Lemon-Dill Sauce and Roasted Vegetables

Recipe:

1. Bake 4 oz salmon fillet at 400°F for 12-15 minutes.

2. Mix 1 tbsp Greek yogurt with lemon juice and dill for sauce.

3. Roast 1 cup mixed vegetables (zucchini, carrots, onions) at 400°F for 20 minutes.

Macros: 340 calories, 35g protein, 20g carbs, 16g fat

Day 18

Breakfast: Vegetable Omelet with Whole Grain Toast

Recipe:

1. Whisk 2 eggs and cook in a non-stick pan with 1/4 cup mixed vegetables (spinach, tomatoes, onions).

2. Serve with 1 slice whole grain toast.

Macros: 280 calories, 20g protein, 20g carbs, 16g fat

Lunch: Mediterranean Wrap with Hummus and Falafel

Recipe:

1. Spread 2 tbsp hummus on a whole wheat tortilla.

2. Add 2 small homemade or store-bought falafel balls, 1/4 cup diced cucumber, and 1/4 cup diced tomatoes.

3. Roll up and serve.

Macros: 320 calories, 15g protein, 45g carbs, 12g fat

Dinner: Lean Beef Stir-Fry with Mixed Vegetables

Recipe:

1. Stir-fry 3 oz lean beef strips with 1 cup mixed vegetables (bell peppers, broccoli, carrots) in 1 tsp oil.

2. Season with garlic, ginger, and low-sodium soy sauce.

3. Serve over 1/4 cup cooked brown rice.

Macros: 350 calories, 30g protein, 35g carbs, 12g fat

Day 19

Breakfast: Overnight Oats with Apples and Cinnamon

Recipe:

1. Mix 1/3 cup rolled oats with 1/2 cup unsweetened almond milk and 1/4 tsp cinnamon.

2. Refrigerate overnight.

3. In the morning, top with 1/2 diced apple and 1 tbsp chopped walnuts.

Macros: 290 calories, 10g protein, 45g carbs, 10g fat

Lunch: Spinach and Mushroom Quiche (crustless)

Recipe:

1. Whisk 2 eggs with 2 tbsp milk.

2. Mix in 1/2 cup chopped spinach and 1/4 cup sliced mushrooms.

3. Pour into a small baking dish and bake at 375°F for 20-25 minutes.

Macros: 200 calories, 16g protein, 8g carbs, 14g fat

Dinner: Grilled Chicken Kabobs with Tzatziki and Greek Salad

Recipe:

1. Grill 4 oz chicken breast, cubed, on skewers with bell peppers and onions.

2. Serve with 2 tbsp tzatziki sauce.

3. Side salad: 1 cup mixed greens, 1/4 cup diced cucumber, 1/4 cup diced tomatoes, 1 tbsp feta cheese, dressed with 1 tsp olive oil and lemon juice.

Macros: 340 calories, 40g protein, 15g carbs, 16g fat

Day 20

Breakfast: Whole Grain Waffle with Greek Yogurt and Berries

Recipe:

1. Toast 1 whole grain waffle.

2. Top with 1/4 cup Greek yogurt and 1/2 cup mixed berries.

Macros: 260 calories, 15g protein, 35g carbs, 8g fat

Lunch: Lentil and Vegetable Soup with Whole Grain Roll

Recipe:

1. Heat 1 cup prepared lentil and vegetable soup.

2. Serve with 1 small whole grain roll.

Macros: 280 calories, 14g protein, 45g carbs, 6g fat

Dinner: Baked Cod with Tomato and Olive Tapenade, Quinoa

Recipe:

1. Bake 4 oz cod fillet at 375°F for 15 minutes.

2. Top with 2 tbsp homemade tomato and olive tapenade.

3. Serve with 1/4 cup cooked quinoa and 1 cup steamed broccoli.

Macros: 320 calories, 35g protein, 30g carbs, 8g fat

Certainly, I'll continue with the next set of days in the same detailed format.

Day 21

Breakfast: Scrambled Tofu with Vegetables

Recipe:

1. Crumble 4 oz firm tofu and sauté with 1/4 cup each of diced bell peppers and spinach.

2. Season with turmeric, garlic powder, and salt.

3. Serve with 1 slice whole grain toast.

Macros: 280 calories, 20g protein, 25g carbs, 14g fat

Lunch: Turkey and Avocado Lettuce Wraps

Recipe:

1. Layer 3 oz sliced turkey breast, 1/4 sliced avocado, 2 slices tomato on 2 large lettuce leaves.

2. Roll up and secure with toothpicks if needed.

Macros: 260 calories, 25g protein, 10g carbs, 15g fat

Dinner: Slow Cooker Chicken Cacciatore with Zucchini Noodles

Recipe:

1. In a slow cooker, combine 4 oz chicken breast, 1/2 cup diced tomatoes, 1/4 cup sliced bell peppers, 1/4 cup sliced mushrooms, and Italian herbs.

2. Cook on low for 6-8 hours.

3. Serve over 1 cup spiralized zucchini noodles.

Macros: 320 calories, 35g protein, 20g carbs, 10g fat

Day 22

Breakfast: Greek Yogurt Parfait with Granola and Fruit

Recipe:

1. Layer 1/2 cup Greek yogurt with 1/4 cup low-fat granola and 1/2 cup mixed berries.

Macros: 290 calories, 20g protein, 40g carbs, 6g fat

Lunch: Caprese Salad with Grilled Chicken

Recipe:

1. Grill 3 oz chicken breast and slice.

2. Arrange 1 sliced tomato and 1 oz fresh mozzarella on a plate.

3. Top with grilled chicken, fresh basil leaves, and 1 tsp balsamic glaze.

Macros: 300 calories, 35g protein, 10g carbs, 15g fat

Dinner: Baked Tilapia with Roasted Brussels Sprouts and Sweet Potato

Recipe:

1. Season 4 oz tilapia fillet and bake at 400°F for 12-15 minutes.

2. Roast 1 cup halved Brussels sprouts and 1/2 small diced sweet potato at 400°F for 20-25 minutes.

Macros: 330 calories, 35g protein, 30g carbs, 8g fat

Day 23

Breakfast: Whole Grain Bagel with Smoked Salmon and Light Cream Cheese

Recipe:

1. Toast 1/2 whole grain bagel.

2. Spread with 1 tbsp light cream cheese and top with 2 oz smoked salmon.

3. Garnish with capers and red onion if desired.

Macros: 280 calories, 20g protein, 30g carbs, 10g fat

Lunch: Quinoa Tabbouleh with Chickpeas

Recipe:

1. Mix 1/4 cup cooked quinoa with 1/4 cup diced tomatoes, 1/4 cup diced cucumber, 2 tbsp chopped parsley, and 1/4 cup canned chickpeas (drained and rinsed).

2. Dress with 1 tsp olive oil and lemon juice.

Macros: 290 calories, 12g protein, 45g carbs, 8g fat

Dinner: Turkey Meatballs in Tomato Sauce with Spaghetti Squash

Recipe:

1. Mix 3 oz ground turkey with breadcrumbs, egg, and seasonings to form 3-4 meatballs.

2. Bake at 375°F for 20 minutes.

3. Simmer in 1/4 cup tomato sauce.

4. Serve over 1 cup cooked spaghetti squash.

Macros: 340 calories, 30g protein, 25g carbs, 15g fat

Day 24

Breakfast: Spinach and Feta Frittata

Recipe:

1. Whisk 2 eggs with 1 tbsp milk.

2. Sauté 1/2 cup spinach in a small oven-safe pan.

3. Pour egg mixture over spinach, add 1 tbsp crumbled feta.

4. Cook until edges set, then finish under the broiler for 2-3 minutes.

Macros: 250 calories, 20g protein, 8g carbs, 18g fat

Lunch: Black Bean and Corn Salad

Recipe:

1. Mix 1/4 cup black beans (drained and rinsed) with 1/4 cup corn, 1/4 cup diced tomatoes, and 2 tbsp diced red onion.

2. Add 1/4 diced avocado and dress with lime juice and cilantro.

Macros: 280 calories, 10g protein, 40g carbs, 12g fat

Dinner: Grilled Shrimp Skewers with Roasted Vegetable Medley

Recipe:

1. Grill 4 oz shrimp on skewers.

2. Roast 1 cup mixed vegetables (zucchini, bell peppers, onions) at 400°F for 20 minutes.

3. Serve with 1/4 cup cooked quinoa.

Macros: 320 calories, 30g protein, 35g carbs, 8g fat

Day 25

Breakfast: Banana Peanut Butter Smoothie

Recipe:

1. Blend 1 small banana, 1 cup unsweetened almond milk, 1 tbsp peanut butter, and 1/2 scoop vanilla protein powder.

Macros: 280 calories, 18g protein, 35g carbs, 11g fat

Lunch: Chicken and Avocado Salad Sandwich on Whole Grain Bread

Recipe:

1. Mix 3 oz diced cooked chicken with 1/4 mashed avocado, 1 tbsp Greek yogurt, and diced celery.

2. Serve on 1 slice whole grain bread with lettuce.

Macros: 320 calories, 30g protein, 25g carbs, 14g fat

Dinner: Vegetarian Stuffed Bell Peppers

Recipe:

1. Mix 1/4 cup cooked quinoa with 1/4 cup black beans, 2 tbsp corn, and 2 tbsp diced tomatoes.

2. Stuff mixture into 1 halved bell pepper.

3. Bake at 375°F for 20 minutes.

4. Top with 1 tbsp shredded low-fat cheese.

Macros: 300 calories, 15g protein, 45g carbs, 8g fat

Day 26

Breakfast: Whole Grain Pancakes with Fresh Berries

Recipe:

1. Mix 1/4 cup whole grain pancake mix with water as directed.

2. Cook 2-3 small pancakes in a non-stick pan.

3. Top with 1/2 cup mixed fresh berries and 1 tsp maple syrup.

Macros: 270 calories, 10g protein, 50g carbs, 5g fat

Lunch: Mediterranean Chickpea Salad

Recipe:

1. Mix 1/4 cup chickpeas (drained and rinsed) with 1/4 cup diced cucumber, 1/4 cup diced tomatoes, 2 tbsp diced red onion, and 5 halved kalamata olives.

2. Dress with 1 tsp olive oil, lemon juice, and herbs.

3. Sprinkle with 1 tbsp crumbled feta cheese.

Macros: 280 calories, 12g protein, 35g carbs, 13g fat

Dinner: Baked Chicken Parmesan with Zucchini Noodles

Recipe:

1. Coat 4 oz chicken breast in 1 tbsp whole wheat breadcrumbs and 1 tbsp grated Parmesan.

2. Bake at 375°F for 20-25 minutes.

3. Serve over 1 cup zucchini noodles tossed with 1/4 cup marinara sauce.

Macros: 330 calories, 40g protein, 20g carbs, 12g fat

Day 27

Breakfast: Cottage Cheese with Sliced Peaches and Almonds

Recipe:

1. Serve 1/2 cup low-fat cottage cheese with 1 sliced peach.

2. Top with 1 tbsp sliced almonds.

Macros: 250 calories, 20g protein, 25g carbs, 8g fat

Lunch: Tuna Salad Stuffed Tomatoes

Recipe:

1. Mix 3 oz canned tuna (drained) with 1 tbsp Greek yogurt, 1 tbsp diced celery, and 1 tsp diced red onion.

2. Stuff mixture into 1 large hollowed tomato.

3. Serve with 1 small whole grain roll.

Macros: 290 calories, 30g protein, 30g carbs, 6g fat

Dinner: Lentil and Vegetable Curry over Cauliflower Rice

Recipe:

1. Simmer 1/4 cup cooked lentils with 1/2 cup mixed vegetables in 1/4 cup light coconut milk and curry spices.

2. Serve over 1 cup cauliflower rice.

Macros: 300 calories, 15g protein, 45g carbs, 8g fat

Day 28

Breakfast: Veggie-Packed Breakfast Burrito

Recipe:

1. Scramble 1 whole egg and 2 egg whites with 1/4 cup mixed vegetables (bell peppers, onions, spinach).

2. Wrap in a small whole wheat tortilla with 1 tbsp salsa.

Macros: 280 calories, 20g protein, 30g carbs, 10g fat

Lunch: Greek-Style Salad with Grilled Chicken

Recipe:

1. Grill 3 oz chicken breast and slice.

2. Toss 2 cups mixed greens with 1/4 cup diced cucumber, 1/4 cup diced tomatoes, 5 kalamata olives, and 1 tbsp crumbled feta.

3. Add grilled chicken and dress with 1 tsp olive oil and lemon juice.

Macros: 310 calories, 35g protein, 15g carbs, 14g fat

Dinner: Baked Cod with Herbed Quinoa and Roasted Asparagus

Recipe:

1. Season 4 oz cod fillet and bake at 375°F for 15 minutes.

2. Cook 1/4 cup quinoa and mix with fresh herbs.

3. Roast 1 cup asparagus spears at 400°F for 10-12 minutes.

Macros: 320 calories, 35g protein, 30g carbs, 6g fat

Day 29

Breakfast: Oatmeal with Almond Butter and Banana

Recipe:

1. Cook 1/3 cup rolled oats with 2/3 cup water.

2. Stir in 1 tbsp almond butter and top with 1/2 sliced banana.

Macros: 290 calories, 10g protein, 40g carbs, 12g fat

Lunch: Turkey and Vegetable Soup

Recipe:

1. Heat 1 cup low-sodium turkey and vegetable soup.

2. Serve with 1 small whole grain roll.

Macros: 250 calories, 15g protein, 35g carbs, 6g fat

Dinner: Grilled Salmon with Dill Sauce, Roasted Sweet Potato

Recipe:

1. Grill 4 oz salmon fillet.

2. Mix 2 tbsp Greek yogurt with fresh dill for sauce.

3. Serve with 1/2 small roasted sweet potato and 1 cup steamed broccoli.

Macros: 350 calories, 35g protein, 30g carbs, 12g fat

Day 30

Breakfast: Avocado Toast with Poached Egg

Recipe:

1. Toast 1 slice whole grain bread.

2. Spread with 1/4 mashed avocado and top with 1 poached egg.

3. Sprinkle with salt, pepper, and red pepper flakes if desired.

Macros: 270 calories, 14g protein, 20g carbs, 18g fat

Lunch: Quinoa and Black Bean Bowl

Recipe:

1. Mix 1/4 cup cooked quinoa with 1/4 cup black beans, 1/4 cup corn, and 1/4 cup diced tomatoes.

2. Top with 2 tbsp salsa and 1 tbsp plain Greek yogurt.

Macros: 300 calories, 15g protein, 50g carbs, 5g fat

Dinner: Slow Cooker Beef and Vegetable Stew with Whole Grain Roll

Recipe:

1. In a slow cooker, combine 3 oz lean beef cubes, 1 cup mixed vegetables, 1/2 cup low-sodium beef broth, and herbs.

2. Cook on low for 6-8 hours.

3. Serve with 1 small whole grain roll.

Macros: 350 calories, 30g protein, 35g carbs, 10g fat

Each day provides approximately 1500-1600 calories, creating a moderate caloric deficit for most seniors while ensuring adequate nutrition. Remember, it's crucial for seniors to consult with their healthcare provider or a registered dietitian before starting any new diet plan, especially if they have existing health conditions or are on medications.

Summary of the Key Nutritional Aspects of This 30-Day CALORIC DEFICIT Diet Meal Plan designed for Seniors

1. Calorie Control:

   - The meal plan provides approximately 1500-1600 calories per day, creating a moderate caloric deficit for most seniors.

   - This deficit supports gradual, sustainable weight loss while still providing adequate energy for daily activities.

2. Protein Emphasis:

   - Each day includes about 80-100g of protein, distributed across all meals.

   - High-quality protein sources (such as lean meats, fish, eggs, and legumes) support muscle maintenance, which is crucial for seniors.

3. Balanced Macronutrients:

   - Approximately 25-30% of calories from protein

   - 45-50% from complex carbohydrates

   - 25-30% from healthy fats

4. Nutrient Density:

   - Meals are rich in vitamins, minerals, and antioxidants from a variety of fruits, vegetables, whole grains, and lean proteins.

   - This supports overall health and helps compensate for the reduced calorie intake.

5. Fiber Focus:

   - The plan emphasizes high-fiber foods like whole grains, legumes, fruits, and vegetables.

   - Adequate fiber (aiming for 25-30g per day) supports digestive health and promotes satiety.

6. Sodium Moderation:

   - Recipes use herbs and spices for flavoring instead of excess salt.

   - This helps manage blood pressure, a common concern for seniors.

7. Calcium and Vitamin D:

   - Inclusion of dairy products and fortified alternatives supports bone health.

8. Hydration:

   - While not explicitly stated in the meals, staying hydrated is crucial and should be emphasized alongside this meal plan.

9. Meal Timing and Frequency:

   - Three balanced meals per day help maintain stable blood sugar levels and provide consistent energy.

10. Portion Control:

   - Meals are portioned to support weight loss while ensuring nutritional adequacy.

11. Variety:

   - The plan includes a wide range of foods to prevent menu fatigue and ensure a broad spectrum of nutrients.

12. Easy Preparation:

   - Most meals are simple to prepare, considering potential

Weekly grocery shopping list for the 30-day CALORIC DEFICIT Diet Meal Plan

This list covers the main ingredients needed for a week, assuming some staples are already in the pantry. Adjust quantities as needed based on individual portion sizes and preferences.

Week 1

Proteins:

- Chicken breast (1 lb)

- Salmon fillets (1/2 lb)

- Lean ground turkey (1/2 lb)

- Eggs (1 dozen)

- Greek yogurt (16 oz container)

- Low-fat cottage cheese (8 oz container)

Fruits:

- Bananas (1 bunch)

- Mixed berries (1 pint)

- Apples (2)

Vegetables:

- Mixed salad greens (1 bag)

- Spinach (1 bag)

- Broccoli (1 head)

- Zucchini (2)

- Bell peppers (2)

- Tomatoes (2-3)

- Cucumber (1)

- Sweet potato (1)

- Cauliflower (1 head)

Grains and Legumes:

- Rolled oats (1 container)

- Quinoa (1 small bag)

- Whole grain bread (1 loaf)

- Lentils (1 small bag)

- Canned chickpeas (1 can)

Dairy and Alternatives:

- Unsweetened almond milk (1 carton)

- Feta cheese (small package)

Canned and Jarred Goods:

- Canned tuna in water (2 cans)

- Low-sodium vegetable broth (1 carton)

- Marinara sauce (1 jar)

Nuts and Seeds:

- Almonds (1 small bag)

- Chia seeds (1 small bag)

Week 2

Proteins:

- Chicken breast (1 lb)

- White fish (cod or tilapia, 1/2 lb)

- Tofu, firm (14 oz package)

- Greek yogurt (16 oz container)

Fruits:

- Peaches (2-3)

- Mixed berries (1 pint)

- Lemons (2)

Vegetables:

- Asparagus (1 bunch)

- Brussels sprouts (1/2 lb)

- Bell peppers (2)

- Tomatoes (2-3)

- Onions (2)

- Carrots (1 bag)

- Mixed salad greens (1 bag)

Grains and Legumes:

- Brown rice (1 small bag)

- Whole wheat tortillas (1 pack)

- Canned black beans (1 can)

Dairy and Alternatives:

- Parmesan cheese (small wedge)

Canned and Jarred Goods:

- Low-sodium chicken broth (1 carton)

- Salsa (1 jar)

Nuts and Seeds:

- Walnuts (1 small bag)

Week 3

Proteins:

- Lean beef cubes (1/2 lb)

- Salmon fillets (1/2 lb)

- Eggs (1 dozen)

- Greek yogurt (16 oz container)

- Low-fat cottage cheese (8 oz container)

Fruits:

- Bananas (1 bunch)

- Apples (2)

- Mixed berries (1 pint)

Vegetables:

- Spinach (1 bag)

- Zucchini (2)

- Bell peppers (2)

- Tomatoes (2-3)

- Sweet potatoes (2)

- Broccoli (1 head)

- Mixed salad greens (1 bag)

Grains and Legumes:

- Quinoa (1 small bag)

- Whole grain English muffins (1 pack)

- Canned chickpeas (1 can)

Dairy and Alternatives:

- Unsweetened almond milk (1 carton)

- Feta cheese (small package)

Canned and Jarred Goods:

- Canned tuna in water (2 cans)

Nuts and Seeds:

- Almonds (1 small bag)

Week 4

Proteins:

- Chicken breast (1 lb)

- White fish (cod or tilapia, 1/2 lb)

- Lean ground turkey (1/2 lb)

- Greek yogurt (16 oz container)

Fruits:

- Peaches (2-3)

- Mixed berries (1 pint)

- Lemons (2)

Vegetables:

- Cauliflower (1 head)

- Asparagus (1 bunch)

- Bell peppers (2)

- Tomatoes (2-3)

- Cucumber (1)

- Carrots (1 bag)

- Mixed salad greens (1 bag)

Grains and Legumes:

- Rolled oats (1 container)

- Brown rice (1 small bag)

- Whole grain bread (1 loaf)

- Lentils (1 small bag)

Dairy and Alternatives:

- Unsweetened almond milk (1 carton)

Canned and Jarred Goods:

- Low-sodium beef broth (1 carton)

- Marinara sauce (1 jar)

Nuts and Seeds:

- Chia seeds (1 small bag)

For all weeks:

Remember to check your pantry for staples like olive oil, balsamic vinegar, Dijon mustard, low-fat mayonnaise, and various herbs and spices. Adjust quantities based on your specific needs and preferences, and consider any personal dietary restrictions or allergies when using these lists.

For Information and Health Tips, Please follow on Instagram: @PlatinumFitAP

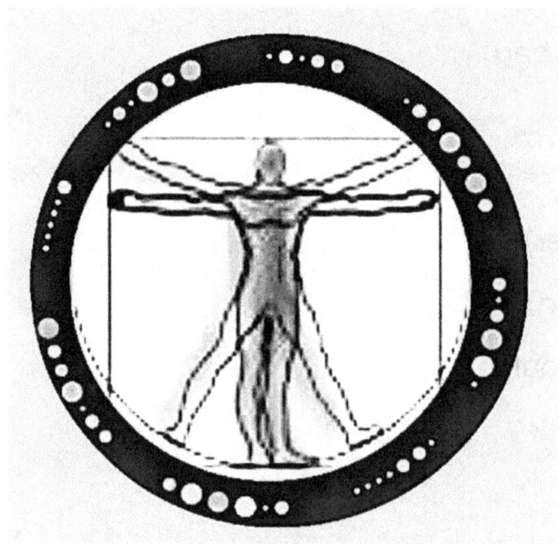